The Essential Lean and Green Cookbook

A Practical Guide to Optimal Weight Loss with 50 Quick and Easy Recipes

By

Spoons of Happiness

policies, processes, or Instructions: contained within is the solitary and utter responsibility of the recipient reader. Under no circumstances will any legal responsibility or blame be held against the publisher for any reparation, damages, or monetary loss due to the information herein, either directly or indirectly.

Respective authors own all copyrights not held by the publisher.

The information herein is offered for informational purposes solely and is universal as such. The presentation of the information is without a contract or any type of guarantee assurance.

The trademarks that are used are without any consent and the publication of the trademark is without permission or backing by the trademark owner. All trademarks and brands within this book are for clarifying purposes only and are owned by the owners themselves, not affiliated with this document.

Table of Contents

Introduction

The Lean and Green diet is quite effective in steady weight loss as it promotes weight loss through the consumption of low-calorie packaged foods, low-carbohydrate home-cooked meals, and personalized training. Basically, it consists of a combination of pre-packaged products called "Fuelings", which have controlled carbohydrates and calories along with lean proteins and non-starchy vegetables. In this way, an intake of 80 to 100 grams of carbohydrates per day is obtained together with a low caloric intake of 800 to 1000 calories.

Gradually replacing the "Fuelings" with a "Lean & Green" meal consisting of balanced meat, vegetable, and a fat meal will allow you to feel satisfied and free of cravings. Once the plan is completed, it is expected that by substituting packaged foods for other lean and green foods, you will adopt better eating habits for life, along with moderate physical exercise and the support of your coach.

What is the Lean & Green diet?

The Lean & Green diet is a weight loss and maintenance plan that combines purchased, pre-packaged foods called "Fuelings" with low-fat, low-carbohydrate home-cooked meals, avoiding the annoying calorie and carbohydrate counting.

The idea is to eat six or more mini-meals a day between fuelings and home-cooked meals. These meals include bars, shakes, crackers, cereals, soup, and mashed potatoes, all of which have soy protein or whey protein as the first ingredient.

The above foods are combined with 3 servings of non-starchy vegetables, 5-7 ounces of lean protein such as tuna, chicken, egg whites, turkey or soy, and no more than 2 servings of balanced fat.

Because carbohydrates are the body's main source of energy, as carbohydrate intake decreases, the body begins to use alternate fuel sources such as protein and healthy fats and the weight loss process begins. Although it may not seem like it, the diet provides a reduced carbohydrate intake.

The Lean & Green diet has several advantages including weight loss resulting from reduced-calorie and carbohydrate intake and portion size control of meals and snacks. The eating plan targets the consumption of 800-1000 calories per day in six specific meal portions. Another benefit is the control of blood pressure by lowering and controlling salt intake. Also, the Green and Lean diet can be maintained over time by avoiding hunger and cravings that make us give up dieting.

In short, lifestyle changes play an active role in our eating habits, leading to eating healthy, exercising more, and reducing stress, and thus living a longer and healthier life.

Chapter 1: Snacks Recipes

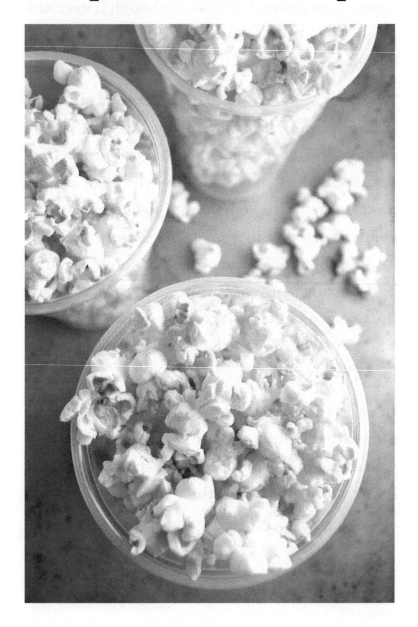

In this chapter, we are going to give you some delicious and mouthwatering recipes on Octavia Snacks recipes.

1. Vanilla Popcorn

(Ready in 20 Minutes, Serve 1, Difficulty: Normal)

Nutrition per Serving:

Calories 90, Protein 1.2 g, Carbohydrates 9.1 g, Fat 5.7 g, Cholesterol 4.1mg, Sodium 50mg.

Ingredients:

- ¼ cup of corn oil

- 1(4 inches) vanilla bean, split lengthwise

- ¾ cup of unpopped popcorn

- 1 tablespoon of superfine sugar

- Salt, to taste

- 2 tablespoons of butter, melted

Instructions:

1. Heat the corn oil for a minute in a large pot over medium-high or high heat.

2. To the oil, add one kernel of popcorn. Pour in the remaining popcorn as well as the vanilla bean as the kernel bursts. Place the pot with a lid and shake softly until the corn begins to pop, then shake vigorously until the popping subsides.

3. Remove from the heat, and dump it into a big tub. Strip the corn from the vanilla beans. Scrape the vanilla bean seeds together and combine them with the honey.

4. Stir in the corn with sugar, salt, and melted butter until evenly coated.

5. Serve and eat.

2. Fruit Leather

(Ready in 6 Hours and 10 Minutes, Serve 16, and Difficulty: Normal)

Nutrition per Serving:

Calories 90, Protein 0.3 g, Carbohydrates 13.5 g, Fat 0.1 g, Cholesterol mg, Sodium 0.8mg.

Ingredients:

- 1 cup of sugar

- ¼ cup of lemon juice

- 4 cups of peeled, cored, and chopped apple

- 4 cups of peeled, cored, and chopped pears

Instructions:

1. Preheat the oven to a temperature of 150 degrees Fahrenheit (65 degrees Celsius). Cover a baking sheet with a sheet of parchment paper or plastic wrap.

2. Combine the sugar, apple, lemon juice, and pear in a blender's container. Cover and blend until smooth. Spread on the prepared pan evenly. Place the pan on the oven's top rack.

3. Bake for 5-6 hours, keeping the door to the oven partway open. When the surface is not tackier, and you may tear it like leather, the fruit is dry.

4. Roll up the plastic wrap and store it in an airtight bag.

3. Grandma Olga's Kolacky

(Ready in 1 Hour and 30 Minutes, Serve 7, Difficulty: Normal)

Nutrition per Serving:

Calories 90, Protein 1.1 g, Carbohydrates 14.1 g, Fat 3.5 g, Cholesterol 12.8mg, Sodium 36.3mg.

Ingredients:

- 1 teaspoon of white sugar

- ¼ cup of warm water (100 degrees Fahrenheit/40 degrees Celsius)

- 2(25 ounces) packages of active dry yeast

- 4 cups of sifted all-purpose flour

- 1 cup of softened margarine

- 4 egg yolks

- 1 cup of sour cream

- 3(10 ounces) of jars apricot or another fruit filling (such as Baker® Fine Dessert Filling)

For Dusting:

- ½ cup of confectioners' sugar

Instructions:

1. In a bowl, dissolve the sugar in hot water, then stir in the yeast. Let stand until a creamy coating of yeast emerges, around 5 minutes.

2. Mix the flour and margarine in another bowl until well mixed, and stir in the egg yolks, one at a time. To make a fluffy but not sticky dough, add in the yeast mixture once incorporated, then stir in the sour cream.

3. Break the dough into 6 same-sized bits, cover with a cloth and refrigerate for a minimum of 1 hour.

4. Preheat the oven to 350 degrees Fahrenheit (176 degrees Celsius). Grease sheets for baking or a line of parchment paper.

5. Rolling out one of the dough balls into 6x8-inch a squared, around 1/8-inch thick, operating on a floured

work surface. Keep refrigerating the other bits of dough.

6. Cut the rectangle into 12 smaller squares, about 2 inches on 1 side, using a pastry cutter or pizza roller. In the middle of each square, put around 2 teaspoons of fruit filling and fold 2 opposite dough corners to meet in the center.

7. To partly enclose the filling, pinch the corners together. Place the filled Kolacky on baking sheets that have been prepared.

8. Bake in the preheated oven for 20-25 minutes, until the cookies begin to become golden brown.

9. Before removing them onto wire racks to finish cooling, let the baking sheets chill for around 2 minutes. Sprinkle Kolacky confectioners' sugar.

4. WWII Oatmeal Molasses Cookies

(Ready in 30 Minutes, Serve 48, Difficulty: Normal)

Nutrition per Serving:

Calories 97, Protein 1.4 g, Carbohydrates 13.5 g, Fat 4.4 g, Cholesterol 7.8mg, Sodium 94.8mg.

Ingredients:

- 2 cups of all-purpose flour

- 2 cups of oatmeal

- 1 teaspoon of baking soda

- 1 teaspoon of baking powder

- 1 teaspoon of salt

- 1 cup of sugar

- ¾ cup of shortening

- 2 eggs, beaten

- 5 tablespoons of light molasses

- 2 teaspoons of vanilla extract

- ½ cup of chopped walnuts (optional)

- ½ cup of raisins (optional)

Instructions:

1. Preheat the oven to 350 degrees Fahrenheit (176 degrees Celsius).

2. Stir the rice, oatmeal, baking soda, baking powder, and salt together in a large bowl.

3. Beat the sugar in another large bowl until smooth and fluffy, and add in the beaten whites, molasses, and vanilla.

4. Mix in the dry ingredients steadily. Stir in the raisins and walnuts. Drop by teaspoonful onto ungreased baking sheets.

5. Bake for 10-12 minutes or until browned slightly. Allow cookies to chill for 5 minutes on a baking sheet before transferring to a wire rack to cool entirely.

5. Grilled Bell Peppers with Goat Cheese

(Ready in 20 Minutes, Serve 6, Difficulty: Normal)

Nutrition per Serving:

Calories 219, Protein 2.9 g, Carbohydrates 2.5 g, Fat 8.1 g, Cholesterol 9.2mg, Sodium 292.3mg.

Ingredients:

- 1 clove of garlic, minced

- 2 tablespoons of olive oil

- ½ cup of goat cheese

- 1 tablespoon of lemon pepper seasoning

Instructions:

1. Core and seed the peppers of the bell. Break each of them into 6 wedges and put them in a resalable bag of plastic Add the garlic and add the olive oil to drizzle. Toss, seal, and set aside for at least 20 minutes to marinate.

2. Preheat a medium-hot outside barbecue and gently grease the grill. In a shallow cup, whisk together the goat cheese with lemon pepper seasoning, and set aside.

3. Cook the peppers until lightly charred, around 3 minutes, on the preheated grill, skin-side-up. Flip over the peppers and spill the cheese carefully onto each pepper. Cover the barbecue lid and cook for 2-3 minutes, before the bottoms are gently charred and even the cheese is warm.

Chapter 2: Breakfast Recipes

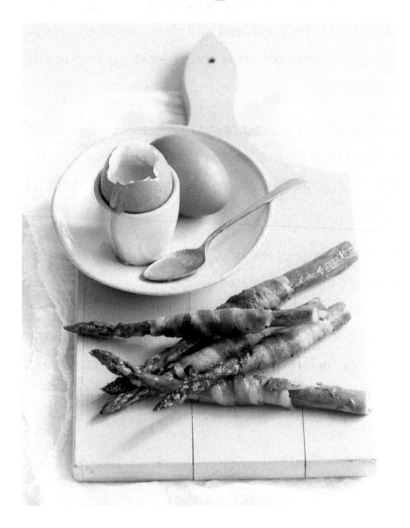

In this chapter, we are going to give you some delicious and mouthwatering recipes on Octavia Breakfast recipes.

6. Asparagus Soldiers with A Soft-Boiled Egg

(Ready in 15 Minutes, Serve 6, Difficulty: Easy)

Nutrition per Serving:

Calories 186, Protein 12 g, Carbohydrates 12 g, Fat 10 g, Saturates 2 g, Sugars 0 g, Fiber 2 g, Salt 0.72 g.

Ingredients:

- 1 tablespoon of olive oil

- 50 g of fine dry breadcrumbs

- 1 pinch each chili and paprika

- 16-20 asparagus spears

- 4 eggs

Instructions:

1. In a skillet, heat the oil, add the breadcrumbs, and then fry until golden and crisp.

2. Season with spices and flaky sea salt, then leave to cool.

3. In a large pan of boiling salted water, cook the asparagus until tender for 3-5 minutes.

4. Boil the eggs at the same time for 3-4 minutes.

5. On a plate, placed each egg in an egg cup.

6. Drain and divide the asparagus between plates.

7. Scatter and serve over the crumbs.

7. Honey Nut Crunch Pears

(Ready in 20 Minutes, Serve 6, Difficulty: Normal)

Nutrition per Serving:

Calories 179, Protein 3 g, Carbohydrates 31 g, Fat 6 g, Saturates 0 g, Sugars 21 g, Fiber 4 g, Salt 0.37 g.

Ingredients:

- 4 ripe pears

- 1 knob of butter

- ½ teaspoon of mixed spice

- 2 tablespoons of clear honey

- 50 g of cornflake

- 25 g of toasted flaked almond

Instructions:

1. Heat oven to 200 degrees Celsius(392 F)/ventilator 180/gas 6. Cut out the core, cut the pears in ½

lengthwise, then top with a tiny butter knob and a sprinkling of mixed spice.

2. Put the pears in a shallow baking dish, then roast for 5 minutes before they start to soften.

3. Meanwhile, in a large microwave bowl, heat the honey and another knob of butter for 30 sec. Toss the cornflakes & nuts.

4. Take the pears out of the oven and then add the cornflake mix to the top. Cook for another minute or before a dark golden color takes over the cornflakes.

5. Allow to cool for a few minutes, then serve warm with ice cream (the cornflakes crisp up again when they cool).

8. Welsh Rarebit Muffins

(Ready in 30 Minutes, Serve 1, Difficulty: Normal)

Nutrition per Serving:

Calories 189, Protein 19 g, Carbohydrates 6 g, Fat 11 g, Saturates 4 g, Sugars 1 g, Fiber 1 g, Salt 0.79 g.

Ingredients:

- 225 g of self-rising flour

- 50 g of plain flour

- 1 teaspoon of baking powder

- ½ level teaspoon of bicarbonate of soda

- ¼ teaspoon of salt

- ½ level teaspoon of mustard powder

- 100 g of strong cheese, half grated and half cubed

- 6 tablespoon of vegetable oil

- 150 g of Greek yogurt

- 125ml of milk

- 1 egg

- 1 tablespoon of Worcestershire sauce

Instructions:

1. Heat oven to 200 C(392 F)/ventilator 180C/gas 6.

2. In a cup, combine the self-raising and plain flour, baking powder, baking soda, salt, and mustard powder.

3. Mix the cheese, grease, yogurt, and sugar, egg, and Worcestershire sauce in a separate bowl.

4. Combine all the ingredients in the muffin tin and divide between the muffin cases.

5. Place for 20-25 minutes in the oven until golden. On a shelf, remove and cool slightly.

6. What you need: ask the children to help prepare everything, weighing scales, measurement bottle, fork, 2 mixing bowls, 12 paper muffin cases, muffin box,

cheese grater, sharp knife, cooling rack, and tablespoon.

9. Hash Browns with Mustard & Smoked Salmon

(Ready in 20 Minutes, Serve 4, Difficulty: Normal)

Nutrition per Serving:

Calories 129, Protein 9 g, Carbohydrates 18 g, Fat 6 g, Saturates 2 g, Sugars 1 g, Fiber 1 g, Salt 1.61 g.

Ingredients:

- 1 large potato (about350 g/12 ounces), washed

- 1 tablespoon of plain flour

- 1 tablespoon of wholegrain mustard or horseradish sauce

- 1 tablespoon of sunflower oil

- 4 slices of smoked salmon

- 1 knob of butter

To Serve:

- Soured cream or crème Fraiche

- Chives

Instructions:

1. On a clean tea towel, grate the unpeeled potato. Bring up the towel edges, and squeeze over the sink to clear the potatoes from any excess water. Place the flour and the mustard or horseradish in a bowl. Season well and combine.

2. Divide the mixture into 8 spheres, then with your hands, flatten it.

3. With the butter and oil, heat a large frying pan, then add the potatoes to the pan.

4. Cook on each side for 2-3 minutes, over medium heat, until golden.

5. On each serving plate, stack a few hash browns and finish with a slice of smoked salmon, a dollop of soaked cream or crème Fraiche, and some chives to serve.

10. Breakfast Smoothie

(Ready in 10 Minutes, Serve 6, Difficulty: Easy)

Nutrition per Serving:

Calories 212, Protein 2 g, Carbohydrates 25 g, Fat 10 g, Saturates 0.1 g, Sugars 24 g, Fiber 5 g, Salt 0.01 g.

Ingredients:

- 1 small ripe banana

- About 140 g of blackberries, blueberries, raspberries, or strawberries (or use a mix)

- Apple juice or mineral water (Optional)

To Serve:

- Runny honey

- Blackberries, blueberries, raspberries, or strawberries

Instructions:

1. In your blender or food processor, slice the banana and add the berries of your choice.

2. Whizz until smooth. Pour in juice or water with the blades whirring to build the consistency you need.

3. Toss on top of a few additional bananas, drizzle with honey and berries, then serve.

Chapter 3: Lunch Recipes

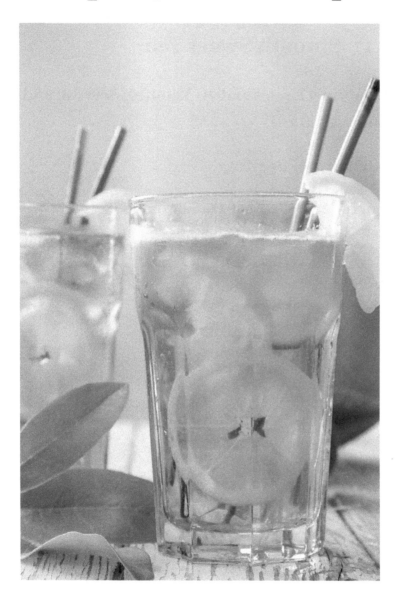

In this chapter, we are going to give you some delicious and mouthwatering recipes on Octavia Lunch recipes.

11. Smooth Sweet Tea

(Ready in 3 Hours and 20 Minutes, Serve 8, and Difficulty: Hard)

Nutrition per Serving:

Calories 127, Protein 0 g, Carbohydrates 18.7 g, Fat 0 g, Cholesterol 0mg, Sodium 41.3mg.

Ingredients:

- 1 pinch of baking soda

- 2 cups of boiling water

- 6 tea bags

- ¾ cup of white sugar

- 6 cups of cool water

Instructions:

1. In a 64-ounce heat-proof glass pitcher, sprinkle a pinch of baking soda. Pour in the boiling water, and then add the tea bags. Cover, and allow for 15 minutes to steep.

2. Remove the tea bags, discard them and whisk in the sugar until dissolved.

3. Use cool water to pour in and refrigerate until cold.

12. Katie's Yogurt Veggie Salad

(Ready in 1 Hour and 50 Minutes, Serve 4, Difficulty: Hard)

Nutrition per Serving:

Calories 311, Protein 8.9 g, Carbohydrates 22 g, Fat 0.4 g, Cholesterol 3.9mg, Sodium 128.9mg.

Ingredients:

- 25 ounces of non-fat plain yogurt

- ½ large English cucumber, halved, seeded, and grated

- 1 carrot, grated

- Salt, to taste

- ½ onion, diced

- ½ red bell pepper, diced

- 1 stalk of celery, diced

- ¼ cup of chopped fresh parsley

- ¼ lemon, juiced

- 1 tablespoon of chopped fresh mint, or to taste

- 2 teaspoons of ground cumin

- Salt and ground black pepper, to taste

Instructions:

1. Spoon the yogurt into a colander lined with cheesecloth and put it aside for at least 30 minutes until most of the water has drained.

2. Sprinkle with salt and put the grated cucumber and grated carrot in a cheesecloth-lined colander. To drain excess water, place a heavy object, such as a bowl, on top of the cucumber and carrot, for 15-20 minutes.

3. In a bowl, mix the milk, cucumber, carrot, cabbage, red bell pepper, celery, parsley, lemon juice, mint, and season with black salt pepper.

4. Refrigerate for at least 1 hour for the flavors to blend.

13. Banana Coconut Idli

(Ready in 45 Minutes, Serve 6, Difficulty: Normal)

Nutrition per Serving:

Calories: 450, Protein 1 g, Carbohydrate 30 g, Fat 0 g, Sodium 0mg, Sugars 19 g.

Ingredients:

For Banana Idli:

- 1 cup of idli batter

- 4 tablespoons of. jaggery powder

- 1 pinch of salt

- 1 pinch of cardamom powder

- ½ ripe banana, chopped

For Coconut Jaggery Cream:

- 1 cup of coconut milk

- 2 tablespoons of jaggery powder

Instructions:

1. For banana idli, add all the ingredients together.

2. Grease with sugar, spoon some batter into the mold, and steam until done. When finished, remove it from the mold.

3. Heat the coconut milk in the jaggery sauce and add the jaggery powder. Stir until dissolved. With warm coconut sauce, serve warm idlis.

14. Summer Squash Salad

(Ready in 25 Minutes, Serve 6, Difficulty: Easy)

Nutrition per Serving:

Calories 197, Protein 3.9 g, Carbohydrate 3.3 g, Fat 19.7 g, Sodium 323.9mg.

Ingredients:

- ¼ cup of white balsamic vinegar

- ¼ cup of lemon juice

- 2 teaspoon of lemon rind

- 2 red chilies

- 2 cloves of garlic, crushed

- 1 tablespoons of olive oil

- 150 g of summer squash(zucchini)

- Sea salt, to taste

- Black pepper, to taste

- Basil leaves

Instructions:

1. Crush 2 cloves of garlic cloves.

2. Now, placed the white balsamic vinegar, lemon rind, red chili, lemon juice, and olive oil in a bowl. Along with sea salt and freshly ground black pepper, add the crushed garlic cloves Blend and mix.

3. Add to the mixture the thinly sliced summer squash and toss to cover it.

4. Keep it aside and leave for 10 minutes to marinate.

5. Place the marinated summer squash and garnish with the baby basil leaves on a serving plate.

15. Sakkarai Pongal

(Ready in 55 Minutes, Serve 6, Difficulty: Normal)

Nutrition per Serving:

Calories: 227, Protein 3.8 g, Carbohydrates 48.7 g, Fiber 1.4 g, Fat 6.9 g.

Ingredients:

- 1 cup of rice

- ¼ cup of yellow moong dal

- 4 cup of milk

- 1 cup of jaggery

- 3 teaspoons of cashew nuts

- 3 teaspoons of raisin

- 5 cardamom nuts

- ¼ cup of ghee

- ½ cup of coconut

Instructions:

1. Soak the rice and cook it with yellow ghee moong dal and mash it properly on a slow flame. Add the jaggery and blend thoroughly.

2. Place ghee in another pan and add cashew nut, raisin, and cardamom. Get it golden, and then add it to the rice mixture.

3. Remove and serve until hot.

16. Freezer Friendly Sandwiches

(Ready in 10 Minutes, Serve 6, Difficulty: Easy)

Nutrition per Serving:

Calories 225, Protein 14.1 g, Carbohydrates 17.0 g, Fat 11.3 g, Saturated 5.3 g, Fiber 1.6 g, Sugars 2.0 g, Sodium 303.0mg.

Ingredients:

- 12 eggs

- 2 tablespoons of milk

- 1 teaspoon of salt

- 1/2 teaspoon of freshly ground black pepper

- 12 slices of cooked bacon, sausage patties, ham, or Canadian bacon

- 12 English muffins

- 12 slices of cheddar cheese, or your favorite cheese

Instructions

1. Preheat the oven at 325 degrees F (165 degree Celsius). Generously oil a 9x13-inch pan.

2. Then mix the eggs, salt, and pepper.

3. Into the greased pan, pour the egg mixture and bake for 18-22 minutes, or only until the center is set. Don't get over-cooked.

4. Remove from the oven and allow to cool into 12 squares before cutting. 4. Top each English muffin with half of the egg, the cheese, the beef, and the muffin with the other ½. If you eat right now, heat the sandwiches for about 5 minutes at 350 degrees or before the cheese melts.

To Freeze:

1. Wrap each sandwich separately in tinfoil, wax paper, or parchment paper and put them in a resealable freezer-safe container. Freeze for a period of up to 1 month.

To Reheat:

1. Thaw overnight in the oven for best results. Cut the paper and wrap a paper towel around the sandwich. Microwave for 40 seconds-Defrost for 1 minute (or 50 percent power). Flip the sandwich over and microwave on high power for 10-30 seconds, until it has warmed through.

2. You can also reheat the sandwiches for around 10-15 minutes in the oven at 350 degrees or in the toaster oven.

Chapter 4: Dinner Recipes

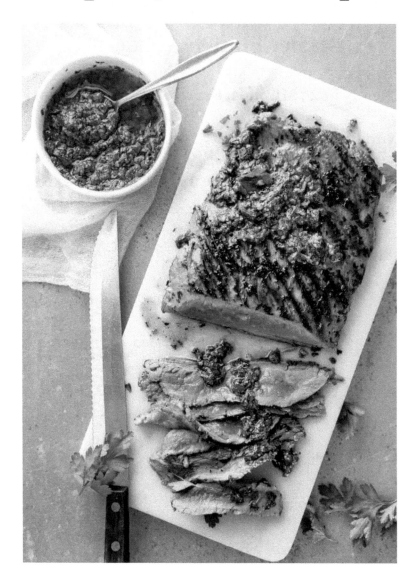

In this chapter, we are going to give you some delicious and mouthwatering recipes on Octavia Dinner recipes.

17. Steak Chimichurri

(Ready in 25 Minutes, Serve 6, Difficulty: Easy)

Nutrition per Serving:

Protein 0 g, Carbohydrates 1 g, Fat 8 g, Cholesterol 0mg, Sodium 15mg, Sugars 0 g.

Ingredients:

- 16 ounces of mixed baby peppers

- 3 tablespoon of olive oil, divided

- 2 12 ounces of strip steaks (about 1 ½ in. thick), trimmed

- 2 tablespoons of red wine vinegar

- 2 scallions, finely chopped

- 1 small garlic glove, grated

- ½ large red chili(seeded), finely chopped

- ½ cup of chopped flat-leaf parsley

- ½ cup of chopped cilantro

Instructions:

1. Heat grill to medium. Toss the peppers in a wide bowl with one tablespoon of oil and ¼ teaspoon of salt and pepper. Season the steak with ½ teaspoon of salt and pepper.

2. Grill steak and peppers, wrapped, sometimes turning peppers until lightly charred and tender, 5-7 minutes. Add the steak and cook until needed, 5-8 minutes on both sides. Transfer the peppers to the bowl and steak to the cutting board and leave for at least 5 minutes to rest before cutting.

3. Meanwhile, mix the vinegar, scallions, garlic, chili, and the remaining 2 tablespoons of oil in a small bowl and pinch each of the salt and pepper. Stir in the parsley and cilantro, add the steak and peppers and serve.

18. Caribbean Chicken and "Rice"

(Ready in 30 Minutes, Serve 6, Difficulty: Easy)

Nutrition per serving:

Calories 370, Protein 37 g, Carbohydrates 37 g, Fat 9 g, Saturated Fat 4 g, Sodium 990 mg, Fiber 10 g.

Ingredients:

- 4 cup of riced cauliflower

- ¼ cup of water

- 4 skinless, boneless chicken-breast cutlets

- 2 teaspoon of olive oil

- ¼ cup of sweetened cream of coconut

- 2 tablespoon of hot sauce

- 2 limes, halved

- 1(15-ounces) can of black beans, rinsed and drained

For Garnish:

- Chopped Cilantro

Instructions:

1. Combine rice cauliflower and water on high for 6 minutes, cover with vented plastic wrap, and microwave.

2. Meanwhile, brush the chicken with olive oil and season with 1⁄2 teaspoon of salt and pepper all over. Grill for 5 minutes on average, turning over once halfway through. Whisk together the coconut sweetened cream and the hot sauce, then brush on the chicken. Grill until cooked through (165 degrees Fahrenheit), brushing and turning 2 more times, about 5 minutes longer. Grill 2 limes, halved, for 2-3 minutes until lightly charred.

3. Toss the black beans and 1⁄4 teaspoon of salt with the cooked cauliflower. Serve chicken with limes over cauliflower, garnished with chopped cilantro.

19. Salmon with Grapefruit and Lentil Salad

(Ready in 15 Minutes, Serve 4, Difficulty: Easy)

Nutrition per Serving:

Calories 330, Protein 36 g, Carbohydrate 22 g, Fat 10.5 g, Saturated Fat 2 g, Sodium 275mg, Fiber 9 g.

Ingredients:

- 2 tablespoon of olive oil, divided

- 567 gramsof skinless salmon fillet

- Kosher salt and pepper

- 2 tablespoons of red wine vinegar

- 1 15-ounce can of lentils, rinsed

- 1 small English cucumber, cut into pieces

- 1 pink grapefruit, peel and pith removed, cut into pieces

- 4 small radishes, thinly sliced

- 6 cups of arugula

Instructions:

1. Heat 1 tablespoon of oil in a medium-sized non-stick skillet. Slice the salmon into 4 parts and season each with 1⁄4 teaspoon of salt and pepper. Cook for approximately 7 minutes, until golden brown. Turn over the salmon and continue to cook until just opaque, about 2 more minutes.

2. Meanwhile, whisk together the vinegar and the remaining tablespoon of oil in a large bowl. Add lentils and coat with a flip.

3. Then mix the grapefruit, cucumber, and radishes. Using arugula to fold and serve with salmon.

20. Grilled Asparagus and Shiitake Tacos

(Ready in 20 Minutes, Serve 6, Difficulty: Easy)

Nutrition per serving:

Calories 350, Protein 7 g, Carbohydrate 36 g, Fat 21 g, Saturated Fat 2 g, Sodium 445mg.

Ingredients:

- 3 tablespoons of canola oil

- 4 gloves of garlic, crushed with press

- 1 teaspoon of ground chipotle chile

- ½ teaspoon of kosher salt

- 8 ounces of shiitake mushrooms, stems discarded

- 1 bunch green onions, trimmed

- 8 corn tortillas, warmed

- 1 cup of homemade or prepared guacamole

- Lime wedges

- Cilantro sprigs

For Serving:

- Hot sauce

Instructions:

1. Heat grill on medium. Mix the oil, garlic, chipotle, and salt in a large baking dish. Toss to coat with asparagus, shiitakes, and green onions. Grill asparagus for 5-6 minutes until tender and lightly charred, turning occasionally. Grill the shiitakes and green onions for 4-5 minutes until lightly charred, turning occasionally. Place the vegetables on the cutting board.

2. "Cut 2" lengths of asparagus and green onions and sliced shiitakes. Serve with tortillas of maize, guacamole, and wedges of lime, cilantro, and hot sauce.

21. Mediterranean Baked Cod

(Ready in 20 Minutes, Serve 4, Difficulty: Easy)

Nutrition per Serving (without rolls):

Calories 220, Protein 32 g, Carbohydrate 8 g, Fat 5 g, Saturated Fat 1 g, Sodium 115mg.

Ingredients:

- 1 medium onion, thinly sliced

- 6 ounces of mini sweet peppers

- Salt

- 1 tablespoon of extra-virgin olive oil

- 1 pot of grape tomatoes, halved

- 8 sprigs fresh thyme

- 680 grams of cod fillets

- ¼ cup of water

- Pepper

For Serving:

- Whole-grain rolls

Instructions:

1. Cook onions, peppers, and 1⁄4 teaspoon salt in olive oil in a 7-8-quart wide-bottomed oven-safe medium-high saucepan for 5 minutes or until onions are almost tender, stirring occasionally.

2. Add the tomatoes and thyme and cook for 2 minutes. Add the cod fillets and broth, and add 1⁄4 teaspoon of salt and pepper to the cod. Cover and bake for 15 minutes, or until the cod is baked, at 450 degrees Fahrenheit (232 Celsius). Discard the thyme sprigs. Serve with whole-grain rolls.

22. Roasted Shrimp & Poblano Salad

(Ready in 35 Minutes, Serve 6, Difficulty: Easy)

Nutrition per Serving:

Calories 201, Protein 17 g, Carbohydrate 9 g, Fat 12 g, Saturated Fat 2 g, Sodium 940mg.

Ingredients:

- 2 medium shallots

- 3 poblano peppers

- 1 tablespoon of canola oil

- 2 teaspoons of chili powder

- 4 radishes

- 1 lime

- 1 avocado

- 453 gramsof large shelled, deveined shrimp

- 1 5-ounce of container mixed greens

Instructions:

1. Heat the oven to 450 degrees Fahrenheit (232 Celsius). Medium shallots in slice 2. Remove the three poblano peppers from the seeds, then slice them.

2. Mix the shallots and poblano peppers with 1 tablespoon of canola oil and 2 teaspoons of chili powder on the baking sheet. 20 minutes to roast.

3. Slice 4 radishes and slice 1 avocado thinly. Only set aside. Squeeze 3 tablespoons of juice out of 1 lime and set it aside.

4. Add 453 g of large shelled, deveined shrimp to the baking sheet after the peppers have been in the oven for 20 minutes. Place it back in the oven and roast for 5 minutes. Slightly cool.

5. Combine the shrimp mixture with the sliced radishes, lime juice, 1/2 teaspoon salt, and 1/5-ounce container of mixed greens when ready to serve. On top, add the sliced avocado.

Chapter 5: Soups Recipes

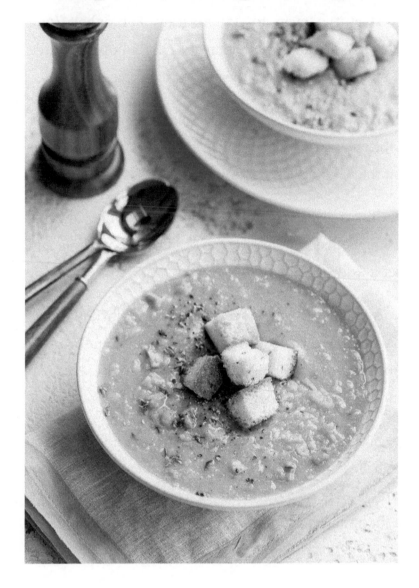

In this chapter, we are going to give you some delicious and mouthwatering recipes on Octavia Soups recipes.

23. Ham and Split Pea Soup Recipe-A Great Soup

(Ready in 1 Hour and 50 Minutes, Serve 8, Difficulty: Hard)

Nutrition per Serving:

Calories 237, Protein 25.1 g, Carbohydrates 37 g, Fat 14.4 g, Cholesterol 39.8mg, Sodium 1186.7mg.

Ingredients:

- 2 tablespoons of butter

- ½ onion, diced

- 2 ribs of celery, diced

- 3 cloves of garlic, sliced

- 453 g of diced ham

- 1 bay leaf

- 453 g of dried split peas

- 1 quart of chicken stock

- 2 ½ cups of water

- Salt and ground black pepper, to taste

Instructions:

1. Place the butter over medium-low heat in a large soup pot. Add the cabbage, celery, and sliced garlic and stir. Slowly cook until the onions, 5-8 minutes, are translucent but not brown.

2. Mix the ham, bay leaf, and split peas together. Sprinkle with chicken stock and water. Stir to mix, and cook gently, about 1 hour and 15 minutes, until the peas are soft and the soup is thick. Occasionally stir.

3. To serve, season with salt and black pepper.

24. Carrot and Ginger Soup

(Ready in 55 Minutes, Serve 6, Difficulty: Normal)

Nutrition per Serving:

Calories 246, Protein 3.5 g, Carbohydrates 33.8 g, Fat 12.8 g, Cholesterol 20.4mg, Sodium 171.7mg.

Ingredients:

- ½ medium butternut squash

- 2 tablespoons of olive oil

- 1 onion, diced

- 453 g of carrots, peeled and diced

- 3 cloves of garlic, crushed or to taste

- 1(2 inches) piece of fresh ginger, peeled and thinly sliced

- 4 cups of water

- Salt and pepper, to taste

- 1 pinch of ground cinnamon

- ¼ cup of heavy cream (Optional)

Instructions:

1. The oven should be preheated to 350 degrees Fahrenheit (176 degrees Celsius). Scoop the seeds from ½ of the butternut squash and place the cut side down on a greased baking sheet. Bake in the oven for 30-40 minutes or until tender. Allow to cool, then with a large spoon, scoop the squash flesh out of the skin and set aside. Discard the skin.

2. Over medium heat, heat the olive oil in a large saucepan or soup pot. Add the chopped onion and garlic and cook until the onion is translucent, stirring well. Add the squash, carrots, and ginger and pour in the water. Bring to a boil and cook until the carrots and ginger are tender, for at least 20 minutes or until tender.

3. In a mixer, or with an immersion blender, purée the mixture. If necessary, add boiling water to thin it but keep in mind that this is meant to be a thick creamy

soup. Send the soup back to the tub, and heat through it. Use salt, pepper, and cinnamon to season.

4. Ladle into serving bowls and as a garnish, if desired, pour a small swirl of cream over the end.

25. Beef Noodle Soup

(Ready in 50 Minutes, Serve 6, Difficulty: Normal)

Nutrition per Serving:

Calories 377, Protein 25.5 g, Carbohydrates 24.8 g, Fat 19.4 g 3, Cholesterol 89.3mg 3, Sodium 1039.7mg.

Ingredients:

- 453 g of cubed beef stew meat

- 1 cup of chopped onion

- 1 cup of chopped celery

- ¼ cup of beef bouillon granules

- ¼ teaspoon of dried parsley

- 1 pinch of ground black pepper

- 1 cup of chopped carrots

- 5 ¾ cups of water

- 2 ½ cups of frozen egg noodles

Instructions:

1. Sauté the stew beef, onion, and celery in a large saucepan over medium-high heat for 5 minutes or until the meat is browned on all sides.

2. Add the bouillon, parsley, carrots, ground black pepper, and pasta with water and eggs. Bring it to a boil, bring it to low heat, and cook for 30 minutes.

26. Squash and Apple Soup

(Ready in 35 Minutes, Serve 6, Difficulty: Easy)

Nutrition per Serving:

Calories 140, Protein 3.1 g, Carbohydrates 28.6 g, Fat 2.8 g, Cholesterol 4.8mg, Sodium 31.8mg.

Ingredients:

- 2 teaspoons of butter

- 1 onion, chopped

- 453 g of butternut squash, peeled and chopped

- 2 apples, peeled and chopped

- 1 small potato, peeled and chopped

- 1 teaspoon of grated fresh ginger root

- 1 pinch of white pepper

- 4 cups of water

- ¼ cup of apple cider

- 1 teaspoon of packed brown sugar

- ½ cup of plain yogurt

- 1 tablespoon of finely chopped toasted pecans

Instructions:

1. Cook the stew beef, onion, and celery in a large saucepan over medium-high heat for 5 minutes or until the meat is browned on all sides.

2. Add the bouillon, parsley, carrots, ground black pepper, and pasta with water and eggs.

3. Bring it to a boil, bring it to low heat, and cook for 30 minutes.

27. Butternut Squash Soup

(Ready in 1 Hour, Serve 6, Difficulty: Normal)

Nutrition per Serving:

Calories 230, Protein 6.9 g, Carbohydrates 59.7 g, Fat 6.8 g, Cholesterol 20.9mg, Sodium 1151.4mg

Ingredients:

- 2 tablespoons of butter

- 1 small onion, chopped

- 1 stalk of celery, chopped

- 1 medium carrot, chopped

- 2 medium potatoes, cubed

- 1 medium butternut squash, peeled, seeded, and cubed

- 1(32 fluid ounces) container of chicken stock

- Salt and freshly ground black pepper, to taste

Instructions:

1. In a large pot, melt the butter and fry the onion, potatoes, celery, carrot, and squash for 5 minutes, or until lightly browned. To cover the vegetables, add plenty of chicken stock. Bring it to a boil. Reduce the flame, cover the pot, and simmer for 40 minutes or until all the vegetables are tender.

2. In a blender, pass the soup and blend until creamy.

3. To achieve the desired consistency, return to the pot and blend in any remaining stock. With salt and pepper, season.

28. Caramelized Butternut Squash Soup

(Ready in 50 Minutes, Serve 1, Difficulty: Normal)

Nutrition per Serving:

Calories 189, Protein 2.9 g, Carbohydrates 24.9 g, Fat 10.3 g, Cholesterol 22.9mg, Sodium 788.4mg.

Ingredients:

- 3 tablespoons of extra-virgin olive oil

- 1360 g of butternut squash, peeled and cubed

- 1 large onion, sliced

- 3 tablespoons of butter

- 1 tablespoon of sea salt

- 1 teaspoon of freshly-cracked white pepper

- 4 cups of chicken broth, or more as needed

- ¼ cup of honey

- ½ cup of heavy whipping cream

- 1 pinch of ground nutmeg, or more to taste

- Salt, to taste

- Ground white pepper, to taste

Instructions:

1. In a large pot, heat olive oil over high heat. Cook and stir the squash until thoroughly browned, about 10 minutes, in hot oil. Stir in the squash onion, sugar, sea salt, and cracked white pepper, cook and stir until the onions are fully tender and begin to brown for about 10 minutes.

2. Over the mixture, add chicken broth and honey, bring to a boil, reduce heat to medium-low and simmer for around 5 minutes until the squash is tender.

3. Pour the mixture no more than half full into a blender. Cover and keep the lid in place and pulse a few times before mixing. In batches, purée until smooth.

4. Stir in the soup to serve with the milk, nutmeg, cinnamon, and ground white pepper.

Chapter 6: Vegan Recipes

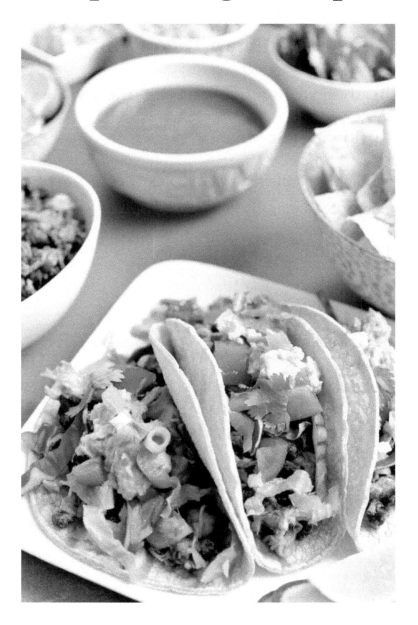

In this chapter we are going to give you some delicious and mouthwatering recipes on Octavia Vegan recipes.

29. Vegan Bean Taco Filling

(Ready in 30 Minutes, Serve 8, Difficulty: Easy)

Nutrition per Serving:

Calories 142, Protein 7.5 g, Carbohydrates 14 g, Fat 2.5 g, Cholesterol 0mg, Sodium 596.3mg.

Ingredients:

- 1 tablespoon of olive oil

- 1 onion, diced

- 2 cloves of garlic, minced

- 1 bell pepper, chopped

- 2(14.5 ounces) cans of black beans, rinsed, drained, and mashed

- 2 tablespoons of yellow cornmeal

- 1 ½ tablespoon of cumin

- 1 teaspoon of paprika

- 1 teaspoon of cayenne pepper

- 1 teaspoon of chili powder

- 1 cup of salsa

Instructions:

1. Heat olive oil over low heat in a medium skillet. Stir in the cabbage, bell pepper, and garlic, and fry until tender. Stir in the beans and mash.

2. Put some cornmeal. Mix the paprika, cayenne, salsa, and chili powder. Cover it, then simmer for 5 minutes.

30. Meyer Lemon Avocado Toast

(Ready in 13 Minutes, Serve 4, Difficulty: Easy)

Nutrition per Serving:

Calories 272, Protein 3.6 g, Carbohydrates 11.8 g, Fat 1.2 g, Cholesterol 0mg, Sodium 270.7mg.

Ingredients:

- 2 slices of whole-grain bread

- ½ avocado

- 2 tablespoons of chopped fresh cilantro, or more to taste

- 1 teaspoon of Meyer lemon juice, or to taste

- ¼ teaspoon of Meyer lemon zest

- 1 pinch of cayenne pepper

- 1 pinch of fine sea salt

- ¼ teaspoon of chia seeds

Instructions:

1. Toast slices of bread to the perfect thickness, for 3-5 minutes.

2. Stir in the cilantro, Meyer lemon juice, Meyer lemon zest, cayenne pepper, and sea salt, and mix the avocado in a dish.

Spread the combination of avocado onto the toast and finish with chia seeds.

31. Slow Cooker Vegetarian Curry

(Ready in 5 Hours and 15 Minutes, Serve 6, and Difficulty: Hard)

Nutrition per Serving:

Calories 124, Protein 6.7 g, Carbohydrates 32.1 g, Fat 0.7 g, Cholesterol 0mg, Sodium 44.6mg.

Ingredients:

- 1 head of cauliflower, chopped

- 1 ½ cups of green peas

- 3 potatoes, chopped

- 3 tomatoes, chopped

- 1 cup of water

- 1 ½ teaspoon of ground cumin

- 1 teaspoon of curry powder

- ¾ teaspoon of ground turmeric

- ½ teaspoon of chili powder

Instructions:

1. In a slow cooker, blend the cauliflower, peas, potatoes, onions, water, curry powder, turmeric, and chili powder.

2. Cook until vegetables are tender, 5-6 hours. Cook on medium heat.

32. Veggie Bagel Sandwich

(Ready in 15 Minutes, Serve 4, Difficulty: Easy)

Nutrition per Serving:

Calories 234, Protein 14.3 g, Carbohydrates 63.7 g, Fat 2.9 g, Cholesterol 0mg, Sodium 680.9mg.

Ingredients:

- 1 bagel, sliced in half

- 1 tablespoon of coarse-grain brown mustard

- 1 leaf of romaine lettuce

- 2(1/4 inch-thick) rings green bell pepper

- 4 slices of cucumber

- 2 slices of tomato

- Salt and freshly ground black pepper, to taste

- 2 slices of red onion

- ½ cup of alfalfa sprouts

Instructions:

1. Spread mustard over the bagel's sliced edges. Layer 1 ½ with the cabbage, green pepper, cucumber, and tomato.

2. Season the tomatoes with pepper and salt. Top with sprouts of onion and alfalfa, then fill with the remaining ½ bagel.

33. Cabbage and Rice

(Ready in 35 Minutes, Serve 8, Difficulty: Easy)

Nutrition per Serving:

Calories 150, Protein 4.2 g, Carbohydrates 30.4 g, Fat 1.6 g, Cholesterol 0mg, Sodium 249.9mg.

Ingredients:

- 1 cup of long-grain white rice

- 2 cups of water

- 2 teaspoons of olive oil

- 1 medium onion, chopped

- 1 clove of garlic, crushed

- 1 head of cabbage, cored and shredded

- 1(14.5 ounces) can of diced tomatoes

- ½ cup of jalapeno pepper rings

Instructions:

1. Combine the rice and water in a saucepan. Bring it to a boil. Cover and minimize to the low heat. Simmer for 15-20 minutes until the rice is tender and water is absorbed.

2. Meanwhile, in a big kettle, heat the olive oil. Add the onion and garlic, cook and stir for about 3 minutes, until fragrant. Add the cabbage and boil, stirring regularly, for about 10 minutes, until the cabbage is finished.

3. Placed the onions, pepper rings, and cooked rice in the mixture. To mix the flavors, boil for 10-15 minutes.

34. Smoky Black Bean Burgers

(Ready in 55 Minutes, Serve 4, Difficulty: Normal)

Nutrition per Serving:

Calories 128, Protein 7.5 g, Carbohydrates 23.4 g, Fat 1.5 g, Cholesterol 0mg, Sodium 753.5mg.

Ingredients:

- 1 tablespoon of ground flax seed

- 3 tablespoons of water

- 1(15 ounces) can of black beans, drained, rinsed, and mashed

- ¼ cup of panko bread crumbs

- 1 clove of garlic, minced

- ½ teaspoon of salt

- ½ tablespoon of Worcestershire sauce

- ⅛ teaspoon of liquid smoke flavoring

- Cooking spray

Instructions:

1. In a small bowl, mix the ground flaxseed and water. Let it sit for about 5 minutes to thicken.

2. In a bowl, blend the flax mix, black beans, panko bread crumbs, garlic, cinnamon, Worcestershire sauce, and liquid smoke until mixed. Shape the batter into 4 patties and place it on a tray. Chill in the refrigerator for about 30 minutes before set.

3. Spray the cooking spray on a skillet and place the patties in the skillet over medium heat. Cook until browned, about 5 minutes on each hand.

Chapter 7: Meat Dishes

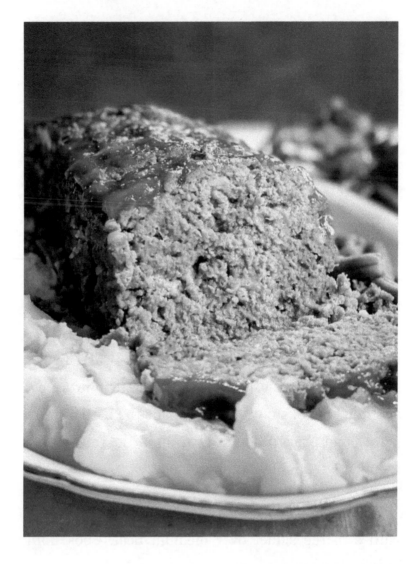

In this chapter, we are going to give you some delicious and mouthwatering recipes on Lean & Green Meat Dishes recipes.

35. Stuffing Meatloaf

(Ready in 55 Minutes, Serve 8, Difficulty: Normal)

Nutrition per Serving:

Calories 289, Protein 19.9 g, Carbohydrates 15.5 g, Fat 15.8 g, Cholesterol 83.5mg, Sodium 429.8mg.

Ingredients:

- Cooking spray

- 680 g of ground beef

- 1 small onion, chopped

- ¾ cup o chicken-flavored bread stuffing mix (such as Kraft® Stove Top®)

- 1 egg

- 1 cup of shredded mozzarella cheese, or to taste

Instructions:

1. Preheat the oven to 400 degrees Fahrenheit (204 degrees Celsius). Use cooking spray to spray a 9x5-inch loaf pan.

2. Heat the olive oil over medium heat in a saucepan, cook and mix the green bell pepper and the onion in the hot oil for 5-10 minutes until the onion is clear and the bell pepper is softened.

3. Add garlic and simmer for 1-2 minutes until it is fragrant.

4. In a large bowl, add ground beef, zucchini, salt, bread crumbs, eggs, carrot, pepper, & bell pepper mixture, using your hands to blend properly. In the prepared loaf tin, press the meat mixture into it.

5. Bake in the preheated oven for 35-40 minutes until it is no longer pink in the middle. A center-inserted instant-read thermometer can read at least 160 degrees Fahrenheit (70 degrees Celsius). Spread on top of the meatloaf with ketchup and bake until bubbling, about 5 more minutes.

36. Mexican Taco Meatloaf

(Ready in 1 Hour, Serve 8, Difficulty: Normal)

Nutrition per Serving:

Calories 227, Protein 21.6 g, Carbohydrates 7.1 g, Fat 16.6 g, Cholesterol 120.2mg, Sodium 468.4mg.

Ingredients:

- 680 g of lean ground beef

- 1 cup of crushed tortilla chips

- ¾ cup of shredded pepper Jack cheese

- 1 small onion, chopped

- 1(1 ounce) packet of taco seasoning mix

- 2 eggs, beaten

- ½ cup of milk

- ¼ cup of mild red taco sauce, or to taste

Instructions:

1. The oven should be preheated to 350 degrees Fahrenheit (176 degrees Celsius).

2. Combine thoroughly in a bowl, season with beef, pepper Jack cheese, tortilla chips, onion, and taco.

3. In a separate bowl, whisk together the eggs, milk, and taco sauce.

4. Add the mixture of meat and stir until well combined.

5. Squeeze the mixture into a 9x5-inch loaf pan and line the middle with a slice of taco sauce.

6. Bake for 45-60 minutes in the preheated oven until baked and browned on top.

37. Tennessee Meatloaf

(Ready in 1 Hour and 55 Minutes, Serve 10, Difficulty: Hard)

Nutrition per Serving:

Calories 223, Protein 17.1 g, Carbohydrates 15.9 g, Fat 11.2 g, Cholesterol 92mg, Sodium 324.1mg.

Ingredients:

- cooking spray

- 1 onion, chopped

- ½ green bell pepper, chopped

- 2 cloves of garlic, minced

- 2 large eggs, lightly beaten

- 1 teaspoon of dried thyme

- 1 teaspoon of seasoned salt

- ½ teaspoon of ground black pepper

- 2 teaspoons of prepared mustard

- 2 teaspoons of Worcestershire sauce

- ½ teaspoon of hot pepper sauce (such as Tabasco®)

- ½ cup of milk

- ⅔ cup of quick-cooking oats

- 453 g of ground beef

- 226 g of ground pork

- 226 g of ground veal

For Brown Sugar Glaze:

- ½ cup of ketchup

- ¼ cup of brown sugar

- 2 tablespoons of cider vinegar

Instructions:

1. Combine the brown sugar, ketchup, and cider vinegar in a cup and blend properly.

2. Preheat the oven to 350 degrees Fahrenheit (176 degrees Celsius). For faster cleanup, spray two 9x5-inch loaf pans with cooking spray or line with aluminum foil.

3. In a covered microwave container, add the onion and green pepper.

4. Until softened, cook for 1-2 minutes. Set aside.

5. Combine the garlic, eggs, thyme, seasoning cinnamon, black pepper, vinegar, Worcestershire sauce, chili sauce, milk, and oats in a large mixing cup. Mix thoroughly. Stir in the green pepper and fried onion. Add ground beef, veal, and bacon. Work all ingredients together until fully blended and uniform with gloved hands.

6. Divide 1/2 of the meatloaf mixture into each prepared loaf pan and pat half of the mixture. Brush the loaves with half the glaze and set aside the rest of the glaze.

7. Bake for 50 minutes in a preheated oven. Take the pans from the oven and drain the fat carefully. Brush the loaves with the glaze that remains. Place them back in the oven and bake for ten more minutes. Remove the pans from the oven and allow the meatloaf to stand before slicing for 15 minutes.

38. The Easiest and Delish Meatloaf Ever!

(Ready in1 Hour and 10 Minutes, Serve 8, Difficulty: Hard)

Nutrition per Serving:

Calories 246, Protein 16.5 g, Carbohydrates 10.9 g, Fat 14.9 g, Cholesterol 76.5mg, Sodium 557.6mg.

Ingredients:

- 1 egg

- 680 g of ground beef

- 1(14 ounces) can of diced tomatoes with green Chile peppers, (such as RO*TEL®), undrained

- 1 sleeve buttery round crackers, (such as Ritz®), crushed

- 1 teaspoon of onion flakes (Optional)

- 1 ½ teaspoon of garlic powder, or to taste

- 1 ½ teaspoon of seasoned salt, or to taste

- ½ teaspoon of ground black pepper, or to taste

Instructions:

1. Preheat the oven to 375 degrees Fahrenheit (190 degrees Celsius).

2. In a mixing bowl, beat the egg and then add the ground beef, tomatoes, and crushed crackers. Season with garlic powder, onion flakes, ground salt, and pepper.

3. Mix until combined equally. Pack into a 9x5-inch loaf pan.

4. Bake in the preheated oven for about 1 hour until the middle is no longer pink. A center-inserted instant-read thermometer can read at least 160 degrees Fahrenheit (70 degrees Celsius).

39. Melt-In-Your-Mouth Meat Loaf

(Ready in 5 Hour and 40 Minutes, Serve 8, and Difficulty: Hard)

Nutrition per Serving:

Calories 328, Protein 24.7 g, Carbohydrates 18.4 g, Fat 16.9 g, Cholesterol 135.6mg, Sodium 841.1mg.

Ingredients:

- 2 eggs

- ¾ cup of milk

- ⅔ cup of seasoned bread crumbs

- 2 teaspoons of dried minced onion

- 1 teaspoon of salt

- ½ teaspoon of rubbed sage

- ½ cup of sliced fresh mushrooms

- 680 g of ground beef

- ¼ cup of ketchup

- 2 tablespoons of brown sugar

- 1 teaspoon of ground mustard

- ½ teaspoon of Worcestershire sauce

Instructions:

1. In a large bowl, combine the eggs, milk, bread crumbs, onion, garlic, sage, and mushrooms. Crumble the ground beef over the mixture and blend to stir properly. Place in a 5-quart slow cooker, then form into a round loaf.

2. Cover and simmer for 5-6 hours before the meat thermometer reads 160 degrees Fahrenheit (71 degrees Celsius).

3. In a shallow bowl, whisk the ketchup, mustard, brown sugar, and Worcestershire sauce with a spoonful of meatloaf sauce. Return to slow cooker and cook on low for around 15 minutes until heated. Let it stand before cutting for 10 minutes.

40. Best Turkey Meatloaf

(Ready in 1 Hour and 15 Minutes, Serve 8, Difficulty: Normal)

Nutrition per Serving:

Calories 296, Protein 19.7 g, Carbohydrates 25.2 g, Fat 13.2 g, Cholesterol 84.5mg, Sodium 880.8mg.

Ingredients:

- 680 g of ground turkey

- ¾ cup of crushed buttery round crackers

- ½ cup of milk

- 1 small onion, chopped

- 1 egg

- 1 ½ teaspoon of salt

- 2 cloves of garlic, minced

- ¼ teaspoon of ground black pepper

For Topping:

- ½ cup of ketchup

- ¼ cup of brown sugar

- 1 tablespoon of Worcestershire sauce

Instructions:

1. Preheat the oven to 350 degrees Fahrenheit (176 degrees Celsius). Grease a jelly roll pan lightly.

2. In a bowl, mix ground turkey, egg, salt, garlic, buttery round cracker crumbs, milk, onion, and black pepper, turn into a loaf, and put on the rolling pan of jelly.

3. In a separate bowl, combine brown sugar, ketchup, and Worcestershire sauce. Set aside.

4. Cook the meatloaf in a preheated oven for 30 minutes, remove the liquid from the oven and rinse. Meatloaf finishes with ketchup topping.

5. Return the loaf to the oven and begin to bake until the middle is no longer yellow, around an additional 30 minutes. A center-inserted instant-read thermometer can read at least 160 degrees Fahrenheit (70 degrees Celsius).

Chapter 8: Salad Recipes

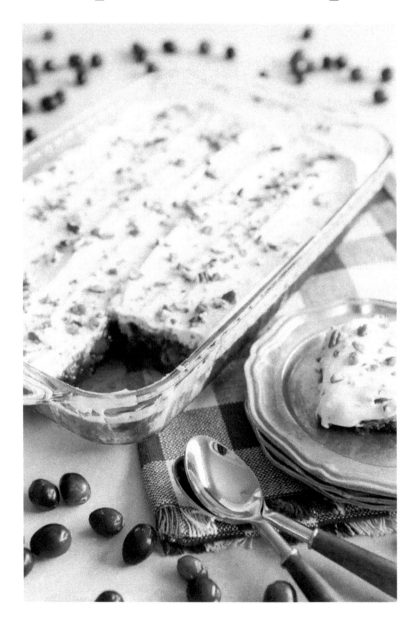

In this chapter we are going to give you some delicious and mouthwatering recipes on Lean & Green Salad recipes.

41. Sour Cream Cranberry Jell-O® Salad

(Ready in 40 Minutes, Serve 24, Difficulty: Normal)

Nutrition per Serving:

Calories 94, Protein 1.3 g, Carbohydrates 14.1 g, Fat 4 g, Cholesterol 8.3mg, Sodium 47.8mg.

Ingredients:

- 1(16 ounces) can of jellied cranberry sauce

- 2(3 ounces) packages of black cherry-flavored gelatin mix (such as Jell-O®)

- 1¾ cups of boiling water

- 1(16 ounces) carton of sour cream

Instructions:

1. In a 3-quart dish, mash the jellied cranberry sauce. Mix the gelatin thoroughly with the cranberry sauce. Pour the boiling water into the mixture and stir for about 3 minutes until the gelatin has fully dissolved.

2. Chill until softly set in the refrigerator, 2-3 hours. Fold the sour cream softly onto the gelatin mixture, leaving the sour cream and gelatin blend in the marbled streaks.

3. Return to the refrigerator until firmly fixed, overnight for 4 hours.

4. Store the leftovers in the fridge.

42. Spinach Pomegranate Salad

(Ready in 40 Minutes, Serve 4, Difficulty: Normal)

Nutrition per Serving:

Calories 273, Protein 9.5 g, Carbohydrates 14.9 g, Fat 21.4 g, Cholesterol 28mg, Sodium 584.6mg.

Ingredients:

- 1(10 ounces) bag of baby spinach leaves, rinsed and drained

- ¼ red onion, sliced very thin

- ½ cup of walnut pieces

- ½ cup of crumbled feta

- ¼ cup of alfalfa sprouts (Optional)

- 1 pomegranate, peeled and seeds separated

- 4 tablespoons of balsamic vinaigrette

Instructions:

1. Place the spinach in a bowl with the salad. Place the red onion, walnuts, feta, and sprouts on top.

2. Sprinkle the top with pomegranate seeds, and sprinkle with the vinaigrette.

43. Roasted Beet Salad

(Ready in 40 Minutes, Serve 4, Difficulty: Normal)

Nutrition per Serving:

Calories 66, Protein 2 g, Carbohydrates 15.1 g, Fat 0.2 g, Cholesterol 0mg, Sodium 136.9mg.

Ingredients:

- 6 medium beets, trimmed and scrubbed

- 2 tablespoons of aged balsamic vinegar

- 2 teaspoons of real maple syrup

- Salt and ground black pepper, to taste

Instructions:

1. The oven should be preheated to 400 degrees Fahrenheit (204 degrees Celsius). Loosely cover the beets in aluminum foil and place them on a rimmed baking sheet.

2. Roast in the preheated oven for 50-60 minutes before quickly pierced with a knife or skewer. Unwrap and cool for about 10 minutes until it is comfortable to handle.

3. Peel and slice the beets into chunks.

4. Stir together the vinegar and maple syrup and season with salt and pepper. Pour the beets over. Refrigerate for at least 1 hour until the beets absorb the flavors. Serve it cold.

44. Pear and Pomegranate Salad

(Ready in 40 Minutes, Serve 2, Difficulty: Normal)

Nutrition per Serving:

Calories 153, Protein 1.6 g, Carbohydrates 23.5 g, Fat 7.1 g, Cholesterol 0mg, Sodium 88mg.

Ingredients:

- 3 cups of green leaf lettuce, rinsed and torn

- 1 Bartlett or Anjou pear

- 1 cup of pomegranate seeds

- 1 tablespoon of vegetable oil

- 2 tablespoons of pomegranate juice

- 1 tablespoon of lemon juice

- 1 teaspoon of prepared Dijon-style mustard

- ½ tablespoon of honey

- Ground black pepper, to taste

Instructions:

1. Divide between two bowls of broccoli. Halve the pear and core it, then cut each ½ of it into slices. Divide and gently combine the pear slices and pomegranate seeds in the two bowls.

2. In a saucepan, blend the vegetable oil, pomegranate juice, lemon juice, mustard, sugar, and pepper. Carry it over high heat to a boil.

3. Reduce the heat and boil until the dressing thickens slightly, stirring regularly for around 2 minutes. Over the salads, pour the warm dressing and serve.

45. Fennel and Watercress Salad

(Ready in 40 Minutes, Serve 20, Difficulty: Normal)

Nutrition per Serving:

Calories 178, Protein 3.1 g, Carbohydrates 8.9 g, Fat 15.4 g, Cholesterol 0mg, Sodium 201.8mg.

Ingredients:

- ½ cup of chopped dried cranberries

- ¼ cup of red wine vinegar

- ¼ cup o balsamic vinegar

- 1 tablespoon of minced garlic

- 1¼ teaspoons of salt

- 1 cup of extra virgin olive oil

- 6 bunches of watercress, rinsed, dried, and trimmed

- 3 bulbs fennel, trimmed, cored, and thinly sliced

- 3 small heads radicchio, cored and chopped

- 1 cup of pecan halves, toasted

Instructions:

1. Mix the cranberries, balsamic vinegar, red wine vinegar, garlic, and salt in a cup. In the olive oil, whisk.

2. Combine the fennel, watercress, radicchio, and pecans in a large salad dish. Stir in the vinaigrette and pour the salad over it.

3. Toss well at once and serve.

46. Chef John's Green Goddess Dressing

(Ready in 40 Minutes, Serve 16, Difficulty: Normal)

Nutrition per Serving:

Calories 124, Protein 0.7 g, Carbohydrates 1.3 g, Fat 13.2 g 2, Cholesterol 10.2mg, Sodium 103.5mg.

Ingredients:

- 1 cup of mayonnaise

- ¾ cup of sour cream

- 1 cup of chopped fresh flat-leaf parsley

- 1 cup of chopped fresh tarragon

- ¼ cup of chopped fresh chives

- 2 tablespoons of fresh lemon juice, or more to taste

- 1 tablespoon of rice vinegar

- 1 anchovy fillet

- 1 clove of garlic, chopped

- 1 pinch of cayenne pepper, or to taste

- Salt and freshly ground black pepper, to taste

Instructions:

1. Mix the mayonnaise, the sour cream, the parsley, the tarragon, the chives, the lemon juice, the rice vinegar, the anchovy fillet, the garlic, the cayenne pepper, and the salt.

2. And black pepper, blend until creamy, in a blender.

Chapter 9: Dessert Recipes

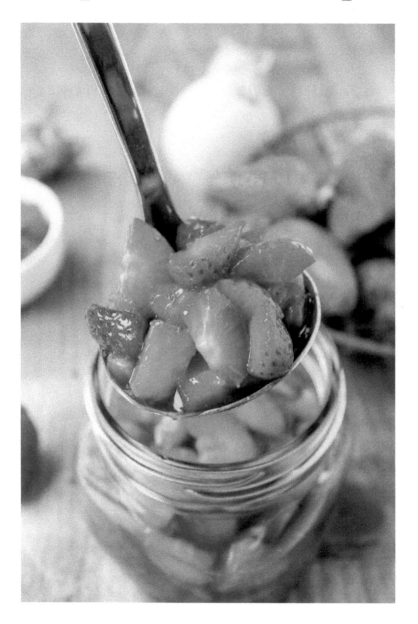

In this chapter, we are going to give you some delicious and mouthwatering recipes

On Lean & Green Dessert recipes.

47. Supreme Strawberry Topping

(Ready in 35 Minutes, Serve 4, Difficulty: Easy)

Nutrition per Serving:

Calories 296, Protein 0.6 g, Carbohydrates 23.7 g, Fat 0.3 g, Cholesterol 0mg, Sodium 1mg

Ingredients:

- 1-pint of fresh strawberries

- ⅓ cup of white sugar

- 1 teaspoon of vanilla

Instructions:

1. Wash strawberries and remove stems, cut large berries in ½ or roughly chop them.

2. Combine strawberries, sugar, and vanilla in a saucepan. Cook over medium-high heat, stirring occasionally. The mixture will sizzle for a while, but then the juice will begin to form. Continue stirring, mash a few strawberries with a wooden spoon or heat-proof

3. Remove from heat. In a blender, puree about 1/3 of the sauce, then mix back into remaining topping. Store in refrigerator.

48. Oma's Rhubarb Cake

(Ready in 1 Hour and 15 Minutes, Serve 12, and Difficulty: Normal)

Nutrition per Serving:

Calories 324, Protein 4.4 g, Carbohydrates 57.7 g, Fat 9 g, Cholesterol 49.6mg, Sodium 252.5mg.

Ingredients:

- 1 ¼ cups of white sugar

- 1 teaspoon of baking soda

- ½ teaspoon of salt

- 2 cups of all-purpose flour

- 2 eggs, beaten

- 1 cup of sour cream

- 3 cups of diced rhubarb

- 1 cup of white sugar

- ¼ cup of butter, softened

- ¼ cup of all-purpose flour

- Ground of cinnamon, for dusting

Instructions:

1. The oven must be preheated to 350 degrees Fahrenheit (176 degrees Celsius). A 9x13 inch baking dish has grease and flour.

2. Stir 1 1/4 cups of sugar, baking soda, salt, and 2 cups of flour together in a big dish. Stir in the sour cream and eggs until creamy, then add in the rhubarb. Pour into the dish that has been prepared and scatter uniformly. Stir the remaining 1 cup of sugar and butter together in a smaller bowl until smooth. Till the mixture is crumbly, whisk in 1/4 cup flour. Sprinkle the mixture softly with cinnamon on top of the cake and then sprinkle it lightly.

3. Bake until a toothpick inserted in the middle comes out clean, about 45 minutes, in the preheated oven.

49. Shudderuppers

(Ready in 1 hrs. 3 Minutes, Serve 20, and Difficulty: Easy)

Nutrition per Serving:

Calories 122, Protein 1.2 g, Carbohydrates 27 g, Fat 1.6 g, Cholesterol 1.4mg, Sodium 59.8mg.

Ingredients:

- 1(14 ounces) package of individually wrapped caramels, unwrapped

- 1(10.5 ounces) package of large marshmallows

Instructions:

1. Build a nice fire and let the wood burn down into coals. This takes about 1 hour.

2. Thread a marshmallow onto a stick, then thread a caramel candy onto the stick in front of the marshmallow. Roast over the coals from the fire until the marshmallow is the desired doneness, but not on fire. Pull the marshmallow up over the caramel so that it is inside. Let cool and enjoy!

50. Smoothie Pops

(Ready in 4 Hrs.10 Minutes, Serve 12, Difficulty: Normal)

Nutrition per Serving:

Calories 39, Protein 1.3 g, Carbohydrates 5 g, Fat 1.8 g, Cholesterol 3.8mg, Sodium 11.1mg. **Ingredients:**

- 1 cup of hulled strawberries

- 1 cup of fresh blueberries

- 1 cup of fresh raspberries

- 1 cup of Greek yogurt

- 5(1 gram) packets of stevia powder

- ½ teaspoon of vanilla extract

Instructions:

1. In a blender, mix the strawberries, blueberries, raspberries, yogurt, stevia powder, and vanilla extract until tender.

2. In 12 ice pop molds, pour the mixture and place sticks or handles. Freeze until firm, approximately 4 hours.

Conclusion

Weight loss and weight maintenance can be easier with the right diet, exercise and the support of a health coach and his or her dietary recommendations. In this case, the Lean & Green diet can be an essential tool to help you lose weight and keep it off because its meals are lower in fat, cholesterol and carbohydrates. Because the foods called "fuelings" are designed with the purpose of being low in calories and carbohydrates and contain the sufficient amount of high quality soy or whey protein required in the daily diet, the Lean & Green diet can be an essential tool to help you lose weight and maintain it.

The "Lean & Green" diet combines meals and a nutritious snack, such as a serving of fruit or a small snack, once the plan is completed, aimed at those who want a higher caloric intake or simply to maintain their ideal weight. For best results, it is recommended to perform low-intensity physical activity for at least 30 minutes, including walking or swimming, or whatever you like, as long as it is done without exaggerated efforts.

It is important to emphasize that the intake of refined cereals, sugary drinks, fried foods and alcohol should be avoided in order to achieve a low intake of carbohydrates and calories, eating only pre-packaged foods and lean proteins and flourless vegetables. Once the target weight is reached, it is expected that the new healthy habits will replace the old ones and a healthy weight will be maintained.

In addition, it is important to emphasize that the support of the coach is essential throughout the dieting process, as well as one's own commitment. For this reason, there is the opportunity to be part of a support group.

Lightning Source UK Ltd.
Milton Keynes UK
UKHW021830010421
381406UK00003B/282